SCIATICA EXERCISES MANUAL

A STEP BY STEP GUIDE ON STRETCHES TO EASE SCIATICA SYMPTOMS

AMELIA CONNER

Table of Contents

CHAPTER ONE

EXERCISES AND SCIATICA: HOW TO DO THEM

Stretches to Ease Sciatica Symptoms

A lot of people ask me, "What is the sciatic nerve?"

The pain from a pinched sciatic nerve can be so severe that you feel like you can't function normally and just want to stay in bed all day. The lifetime prevalence of this condition is between 10% and 40%, so it's likely that you know more than one person who has it.

The sciatic nerve branches off from the buttocks, hips, and lumbar region to travel down both legs before meeting at the ankles and feet. When there is irritation or inflammation along this path, you may experience sciatica.

Common triggers for sciatic pain include:

• a herniated disc

Reduction in the space available for the spinal cord to move (called spinal stenosis)

- injury

It's important to note that piriformis syndrome, another potential source of sciatica, is also a real thing. The piriformis muscle spans the posterior aspect of your spine, beginning at the buttocks, all the way to the anterior thigh. When this muscle spasms, it can pinch the nearby sciatic nerve. The result may be excruciating sciatic pain.

a licensed physical therapist, says there are many potential triggers for sciatica pain. She says that figuring out what is immobile is the first step in fixing the issue. The hips and lower back are frequent trouble spots.

According to Doctors, a certified strength and conditioning specialist, "any stretch that can externally rotate the hip to provide some relief" is the best way to alleviate most sciatica pain.

CHAPTER TWO

Position: pigeon pose (lying down)

Pigeon pose

In the pigeon pose, which involves bending forward,

• Knee to the asymmetrical shoulder

Back stretches while seated

Position: standing hamstring stretch

Simple stretches while seated

Exercise for the piriformis muscle while standing

- a stretch for the groin and the long abductors

To stretch the hamstrings, try the scissor move.

First, the pigeon pose, where you lie back and relax.

One of several pigeon stretches that can aid in stretching the piriformis muscle is the reclining pigeon pose.

The pigeon pose, or reclined bird, is a standard yoga position. The result is a more flexible hip girdle. This stretches in a variety of ways. The first is the reclining pigeon pose, which is a simplified version often used as a starting point. Trying out the reclining position first is recommended when beginning treatment.

First, while still on your back, lift your right leg so that it forms a right angle with the body. Lock your fingers together and clasp your hands behind your thigh.

Then, bring your right ankle over your left knee while lifting your left leg.

Try to maintain the position for a few seconds. The piriformis muscle, which can become inflamed and press on the sciatic nerve, is stretched out in this way, providing relief. All the hip rotator muscles deep tissue are stretched as well.

4. Switch legs and repeat the process.

Once you and your PT have mastered the reclining pigeon pose, you can progress to the sitting and forward versions.

The pigeon pose, where the subject is seated

You can also adopt a cross-legged position to achieve the pigeon pose.

courtesy of Goodboy Pictures/Getty Images

First, get down on the floor and sit up straight with your legs out in front of you.

Second, bring your right ankle over your left knee by bending your right knee.

Third, stoop forward until your upper body touches your lower thigh.

Fourth, maintain the position for 15 to 30 seconds. Both the glutes and the lower back get a nice stretch.

Five, do the same thing on the reverse.

Pose 3: Pigeon in front position

To get into this pigeon pose variation, kneel on the floor with your palms facing the floor.

First, get down on all fours and kneel.

Two, bring your right foot off the ground and forward in front of you. Keep your lower leg flat on the floor at a right angle to your body. Your right knee should remain on the right side of your body while your right foot moves in front of your left knee.

3. Extend your left leg behind you, placing the sole of your foot on the floor and pointing your toes backward.

The fourth step is to gradually transfer your weight from your arms to your legs. Put your hands on your legs and sit up straight.

5, Take a few deep breaths. While releasing your breath, lean forward over your front leg. You should lean on your arms as much as possible.

Six, do it again on the reverse.

The Knee to the Opposite Shoulder Position

One performs the knee-to-opposite-shoulder stretch while lying on one's back.

By relaxing the gluteal and piriformis muscles, which can become inflamed and press on the sciatic nerve, this simple stretch can help alleviate sciatica pain.

One, get on your back with your legs spread apart and your feet flexed up.

2.Bend your right knee and clasp your hands around your shin.

Third, bring your right shin to your left shoulder by gently bringing it across your body.

Don't move it for the next 30 seconds. Don't force your knee any farther than it can go comfortably. Not pain, but a nice, relaxing stretch in the muscle is what you want to experience.

Simply return your leg to its original position by pushing your knee in.

5. Do three sets, and then switch legs.

Stretching the spine while seated

The seated spinal stretch can help alleviate sciatic nerve pressure if you turn to one side.

When the vertebrae in the back become compressed, it can cause excruciating pain radiating down the sciatic nerve. The sciatic nerve is less likely to experience compression thanks to this stretch's ability to open up the spine.

Sit on the floor with your legs spread apart and your feet flexed up.

Second, put the outside of your right foot flat on the floor, bending your knee slightly.

3 Gently turn your body to the right by placing your left elbow on the outside of your right knee.

Four, pause for 30 seconds three times, and then switch sides.

6) Hamstring stretches while standing

To perform a standing hamstring stretch, stand with your right foot propped up on an elevated surface, such as a chair.

Pain and stiffness in the hamstring from sciatica can be relieved with this stretch.

First, raise your right foot to a level above your hips. A chair, an ottoman, or a stair step are all examples. Make sure your toes and leg are completely straight by flexing your foot. Keep a small bend in your knee if it has a tendency to hyperextend.

Secondly, lean forward a little bit to get closer to your foot. As you travel further, the stretch becomes more intense. Don't exert yourself to the point of discomfort.

3. Instead of lifting your hips up, let your raised leg's hips sink. Put a yoga strap or long exercise band around your right thigh and under your left foot to help you relax your hip.

4. Keep this position for at least 30 seconds, then switch sides and do it again.

Preliminary stretches while seated

Keep your back straight as you stretch each leg individually in the basic seated stretch.

Physical Energy Mental Proactivity

To begin, find a comfortable chair and cross your sore leg over the knee of your uninjured leg. Once you're ready, proceed with these measures:

• Lean forward from the hips while keeping your back straight. If you can bend over a little further without discomfort, that is. If it hurts, you should stop.

Hold this position for 30 seconds and then switch legs.

Exercising the piriformis muscle while standing is the eighth move.

In order to maintain stability as you lengthen your piriformis muscle while standing, you can rest your hands on your hips.

Here's another standing stretch that can ease sciatica symptoms. If you're strong enough, you can do this without any assistance, or you can stand with your feet about 24 inches from a wall for added stability.

As you stand, cross your sore knee over the knee of your uninjured leg. Try forming the number 4 by bending your standing leg at the knee and squatting down 45 degrees.

Straighten your back and bend forward at the waist while swinging your arms downward. Tend to that spot for a minute or two.

Repeat with the other leg.

9. A stretch for the groin and the long adductor muscles

Lean forward until you feel a stretch in your groin and long adductor muscle.

This is an Alyssa Kiefer illustration.

To perform this stretch, find a comfortable seated position on the ground and extend your legs as far as you comfortably can in front of you.

• Squat down with your torso slanted downward and your hands on the floor in front of you.

Keep your elbows on the ground and lean forward. Ten to twenty seconds is an appropriate amount of time to maintain the position. If it hurts, you should stop.

Ten. The Scissor Hamstring Stretch

The scissor hamstring stretch is a bending exercise that helps release tension in the hamstrings and relieve sciatica by lowering pressure on the nerve. Stocksy United/Jose Coello

The ischium is a component of the pelvic girdle along with the ilium and the pubis; from it extend the ischial tuberosity, colloquially known as the sit or sitz bones.

With the help of the sacrotuberous ligament, the hamstrings are attached to the ischial tuberosity (STL). Tense hamstring muscles can give the impression of sciatica.

To reduce the strain on the sciatic nerve, loosen your hamstrings with this stretch. Performing this exercise on a regular basis could be beneficial.

In order to do this, step three feet back with your right foot from where you left off with your left foot.

• Lean forward at the hips and back at the shoulders; avoid putting more weight on your right foot. To make an informed decision, perhaps a mirror will help.

Do as I say and rest your hands on your hips. If you feel more secure using a chair, feel free to do so.

Keeping your back straight, bend at the waist and push your torso over your front leg. The front leg should bear the bulk of your weight.

• Hold for 5-10 seconds, and then switch legs and repeat on the other side. Repeat the stretch three to five times for each leg.

CHAPTER THREE

Caution should be taken during exercise.

Kovacs stresses the importance of not assuming you will have the level of flexibility required for the exercises. Don't believe the hype: "Don't think that because of what you see on YouTube or TV that you can get into these positions," he warns. All of the exercise demonstrators are extremely flexible, long-time practitioners.

You should stop immediately if you're experiencing any pain.

a physical therapist at Duke Sports Medicine Center and member of the American Medical Society for Sports Medicine, says that there's no one-size-fits-all exercise for people who have sciatic nerve pain.

She suggests adjusting the positions slightly, such as pulling your knees in more or less, and noticing how they feel. "If one feels better, that is the treatment you want to pursue," she advises.

Martinez says that anyone experiencing even mild sciatic nerve pain for more than a month should see a doctor or physical therapist. They may find relief with an in-home exercise program tailored specifically to their pain.